Facial Gua Sha for Women

A Beginner's Step-by-Step Guide on How to Use the Tool and Overview on its Use Cases for Facial Beauty and Health

copyright © 2022 Felicity Paulmann

All rights reserved No part of this book may be reproduced, or stored in a retrieval system, or transmitted in any form or by any means, electronic, mechanical, photocopying, recording, or otherwise, without express written permission of the publisher.

Disclaimer

By reading this disclaimer, you are accepting the terms of the disclaimer in full. If you disagree with this disclaimer, please do not read the guide.

All of the content within this guide is provided for informational and educational purposes only, and should not be accepted as independent medical or other professional advice. The author is not a doctor, physician, nurse, mental health provider, or registered nutritionist/dietician. Therefore, using and reading this guide does not establish any form of a physician-patient relationship.

Always consult with a physician or another qualified health provider with any issues or questions you might have regarding any sort of medical condition. Do not ever disregard any qualified professional medical advice or delay seeking that advice because of anything you have read in this guide. The information in this guide is not intended to be any sort of medical advice and should not be used in lieu of any medical advice by a licensed and qualified medical professional.

The information in this guide has been compiled from a variety of known sources. However, the author cannot attest to or guarantee the accuracy of each source and thus should not be held liable for any errors or omissions.

You acknowledge that the publisher of this guide will not be held liable for any loss or damage of any kind incurred as a result of this guide or the reliance on any information provided within this guide. You acknowledge and agree that you assume all risk and responsibility for any action you undertake in response to the information in this guide.

Using this guide does not guarantee any particular result (e.g., weight loss or a cure). By reading this guide, you acknowledge that there are no guarantees to any specific outcome or results you can expect.

All product names, diet plans, or names used in this guide are for identification purposes only and are the property of their respective owners. The use of these names does not imply endorsement. All other trademarks cited herein are the property of their respective owners.

Where applicable, this guide is not intended to be a substitute for the original work of this diet plan and is, at most, a supplement to the original work for this diet plan and never a direct substitute. This guide is a personal expression of the facts of that diet plan.

Where applicable, persons shown in the cover images are stock photography models and the publisher has obtained the rights to use the images through license agreements with third-party stock image companies.

Table of Contents

Introduction	**8**
Background and History of Gua Sha	**11**
Gua Sha Around the World	12
Other Names and Modern Popularity	13
Anatomy of Gua Sha Benefits	13
The Gua Sha Tools	**18**
Gua Sha Tools Based on Materials	18
Gua Sha Tool Shapes and Their Applications	21
How to Spot Authentic, High-Quality Gua Sha Tools	23
How do Practitioners Perform the Gua Sha Technique?	**25**
How Often Should Gua Sha be Performed?	26
Uses of Gua Sha	**28**
Treating Pain and Inflammation	28
Boosting Immunity	29
Relieving Stress	29
Relieving Fatigue	29
Relieving Headaches	30
Improving Digestion	30
Treating Flu	31
Detoxifying the Body	31
Relieving Menstrual Cramps	31
For Skincare	32
For the Body	33
Gua Sha for Specific Health Conditions	**38**
Alleviating Tension Headaches and Migraines	38
Managing Arthritis and Fibromyalgia Symptoms	39
Easing Menstrual Cramps	40
Promoting Digestion	41
How Gua Sha Treatment Complements Other Traditional	

Chinese Medicine (TCM) Practices   **43**
    How Gua Sha Complements TCM Techniques   44
    The Role of Meridians and Energy Flow in Gua Sha Therapy 46
    Case studies from TCM practitioners using Gua Sha in treatments.   47

The Risks of the Gua Sha Technique   **49**
    Common Mistakes and How to Avoid Them   50
    Gua Sha Safety Tips: Practicing Safely and Effectively   53
    Is Gua Sha Right for Me?   56

Women and Facial Beauty   **59**

Benefits of Using Gua Sha on your Face   **61**

Facial Gua Sha for Targeted Concerns   **64**
    Reducing Under-Eye Puffiness and Dark Circles   64
    Sculpting the Jawline and Cheekbones   65
    Minimizing Fine Lines and Wrinkles   66
    Performing Gua Sha for Sinus Relief   66
    Stress Reduction with Gua Sha   67

5 Step-by-Step Guide on How to Perform Gua Sha   **69**
    Step 1: Choose the Right Gua Sha Tool for Your Needs   69
    Step 2: Prepare Your Skin   70
    Step 3: Begin Scraping with Proper Technique   71
    Step 4: Final Touch - Cleaning and Cooling   73
    Step 5: Moisturize and Relax   74
    Creating a Gua Sha Routine   75

DIY Gua Sha Recipes for Oils and Creams   **77**
    Why Lubrication Matters for Gua Sha   77
    DIY Recipes for Gua Sha Oils   78
    Anti-Inflammatory Calming Oil   79
    Hydrating Glow Oil (For Dry Skin)   80
    Balancing Facial Oil (For Oily or Acne-Prone Skin)   81
    Brightening Citrus Oil (For Dull or Uneven Skin Tone)   82
    Soothing Recovery Oil (For Irritated or Post-Sunburn Skin)   83

    DIY Recipes for Gua Sha Creams   85
    Gentle Chamomile Cream (For Sensitive or Red-Prone Skin) 86
    Anti-Aging Rosehip Cream (For Mature Skin)   87
    Lightweight Green Tea Gel (For Oily or Acne-Prone Skin)   88
    Brightening Vitamin C Cream (For Dull or Uneven Skin Tone) 89
    Deep Hydration Avocado Cream (For Extremely Dry or Flaky Skin)   90
    Tips for Storing and Using DIY Products   91

Gua Sha and Graston Technique   93
Conclusion   95
FAQ   98
References and Helpful Links   101

Introduction

The term "qi" refers to the energy that circulates throughout the body, as described by traditional Chinese medicine. It is said to be responsible for both a person's bodily and mental wellness. It is believed that the kidneys are the source of qi and that it travels through the body in a network of channels known as the meridians.

It is believed that there are twelve primary meridians, each of which is associated with a distinct organ. According to traditional Chinese medicine, illness results from an imbalance in the flow of qi. Acupuncture, herbal medicine, and gua sha are some of the practices that are utilized in traditional Chinese medicine to bring about a state of balance.

In Gua Sha, a kind of traditional Chinese medicine, the patient's skin is scraped using a tool that is both smooth and curved to stimulate circulation and has a therapeutic effect. It is believed that the technique dates back to the 7th century, and it is being used today for a range of diseases, including the reduction of pain, the prevention of colds and flu, and the treatment of digestive issues.

When doing Gua Sha, a tool made of jade or another type of stone that is polished and curved is often used. After applying oil to the surface of the skin, the practitioner will scrape the instrument in a manner that is both hard and soft over the surface of the skin. The scrape should not be uncomfortable; nevertheless, some patients may feel bruising following the treatment due to the nature of the procedure.

Gua Sha may have a variety of beneficial effects, some of which include the alleviation of pain, enhancement of circulation, reduction of inflammation, and improvement of immunological function. In addition, Gua Sha may be used to treat respiratory illnesses like colds and flu, as well as digestive issues like constipation and diarrhea.

Gua Sha is an effective technique for reducing wrinkles and promoting a youthful appearance. It can also help with menstrual cramps, menopausal symptoms, and PMS.

The frequency of Gua Sha treatments depends on the condition being treated. For general well-being, one or two sessions per week may suffice, while acute issues might require three or more sessions weekly.

When performed by a skilled practitioner, Gua Sha is generally safe, though minor bruising or skin irritation can occur. If you're unsure whether it's right for you, consult a healthcare professional before booking a session.

In this beginner's guide, we'll take a deeper look at the following subtopics:

- Background and history of gua sha
- The Gua Sha Tools Materials and Shapes
- How do practitioners perform the gua sha technique?
- The uses of the gua sha technique
- The gua sha technique in conjunction with the other traditional Chinese medicines
- The risks of the gua sha technique
- Women and facial beauty
- Benefits of using gua sha on your face
- Step-by-step guide on how to perform gua sha on your face
- When to know if gua sha is right for you?
- The gua sha and Graston technique's similarities and differences

Keep reading to learn more about this ancient Chinese healing practice and how it can benefit your overall health and well-being. We'll explore its origins, the tools used in Gua Sha, how practitioners perform the technique, and the various uses of this therapy. By the end of this guide, you'll have a better understanding of Gua Sha and whether it is the right treatment for your specific needs.

Background and History of Gua Sha

Gua Sha, a therapeutic practice rooted in ancient medicine, may date back to the Paleolithic era. Early practitioners used stones or hard objects to scrape the body, relieving pain or even inducing unconsciousness in emergencies. The technique is mentioned in the "Prescriptions for 52 Diseases", a collection of medical manuscripts found in 1973 in the Ma Wang Dui Han tomb in Changsha, Hunan, China. Dating to the Shang-Zhou dynasty (1065–771 BCE), this text is the earliest known record of Chinese materia medica, documenting traditional therapies like Gua Sha.

Today, Gua Sha remains widely practiced in China, continuing its deep connection to Traditional Chinese Medicine while gaining global recognition for its therapeutic and skincare benefits. Its evolution and cultural adaptations across different countries highlight its versatility and enduring appeal.

Gua Sha Around the World

Indonesia:

Known as kerikan or kerokan, Gua Sha is commonly practiced as a household remedy in Indonesia. Rooted in traditional Chinese influences that reached Southeast Asia in the 5th century, kerokan focuses on expelling "cold wind," believed to be the cause of ailments like colds or the flu (referred to as Masuk angin or "entry of wind"). The scraping technique, passed down through generations, remains a popular method for alleviating symptoms of illness.

India:

Introduced to India in the 15th century during Admiral Zheng He's naval campaigns, Gua Sha found a place alongside Ayurvedic medicine. It is thought to purify the body, reduce fevers, and promote relaxation. The practice aligns with Ayurvedic principles, emphasizing improved circulation and the body's innate healing abilities.

Vietnam:

Vietnamese culture integrates Gua Sha under the name co gió, which translates to "scratch the wind." The practice, heavily influenced by Chinese medical traditions, has been part of Vietnam's healthcare system since the 5th–7th centuries CE. Commonly used to treat colds, fever, and body aches, it remains an accessible and trusted remedy in Vietnamese homes.

Other Names and Modern Popularity

Across different cultures, Gua Sha has been given unique local names. English speakers often call it "spooning" or "coining," whereas the French use the term "tribo-effleurage." Each name reflects adaptations of the technique while retaining its essence of scraping or rubbing the skin to bring about therapeutic effects.

Recently, Gua Sha has seen a remarkable resurgence in popularity. With more people turning to alternative wellness practices, it has captured attention for its holistic health benefits and its ability to enhance skin radiance. It is now celebrated as both a therapeutic tool and a beauty ritual, with its simplicity and effectiveness making it a widely embraced practice worldwide.

Anatomy of Gua Sha Benefits

Gua Sha offers restorative effects that span both the physical body and the energetic systems outlined in Traditional Chinese Medicine (TCM). By understanding how it works physiologically, you can appreciate its dual role in promoting scientific and holistic wellness.

1. **Lymphatic Drainage and Detoxification:** Gua Sha supports the lymphatic system, helping the body

remove toxins, excess fluid, and waste by stimulating lymph flow and filtration.

When you glide a Gua Sha tool over your skin, the repetitive, gentle scraping motion helps to:

- ***Boost Lymphatic Flow:*** The tool pushes stagnant lymph fluid toward lymph nodes, ensuring optimal filtration and clearance.
- ***Reduce Puffiness and Swelling:*** By draining excess fluid, particularly in delicate areas like the under-eyes, Gua Sha reduces puffiness and provides a sculpting effect.
- ***Detoxify Skin and Tissues:*** Enhanced lymph movement prevents toxin build-up, leading to clearer, healthier skin.

2. **Improved Blood Circulation:** Gua Sha promotes healthy blood flow by stimulating microcirculation in the small vessels under the skin, helping deliver nutrients and remove waste. Here's how it works:
   - ***Vasodilation:*** The scraping motion signals the tiny capillaries under your skin to dilate, allowing for an increased flow of oxygenated blood.
   - ***Oxygen and Nutrient Delivery:*** Boosted circulation nourishes cells, giving your skin a radiant glow and aiding in the skin's repair processes.

- ***Speeding Up Recovery:*** Enhanced blood flow also clears away inflammatory substances, promoting quicker recovery from muscle tension, swelling, or fatigue.

On a visual level, the temporary redness or slight bruising that may appear post-treatment (known as sha) is an indicator of blood rising to the skin surface, signifying increased circulation and healing activity.

3. **Reducing Cellular-Level Inflammation:** Inflammation is the body's immune response to stress, injury, or infection, but chronic inflammation can cause swelling, discomfort, and long-term conditions like arthritis.

Gua Sha addresses inflammation both in localized areas and across the body:

- ***Breakdown of Cytokines:*** Gua Sha has been shown to reduce pro-inflammatory cytokines—molecules that signal inflammation—helping alleviate swelling and pain at a cellular level.
- ***Tissue Regeneration:*** By stimulating microcirculation and improving oxygen delivery, Gua Sha creates an optimal environment for cellular repair and renewal.

- *Muscle Relaxation:* Gua Sha's massaging action soothes muscle tension, further reducing the inflammatory response caused by tightness or strain in connective tissues.

4. **Energy Flow and TCM Perspective:** In Traditional Chinese Medicine, the body's energy, or qi, flows through a system of pathways known as meridians. Blocked or stagnant qi can lead to discomfort, illness, or emotional imbalance.

Gua Sha works on this energetic level by:

- *Unblocking Energy Stagnation:* The scraping motion stimulates points along the meridians, helping to unblock qi and allowing it to flow freely again.
- *Balancing Yin and Yang:* The technique restores harmony between opposing forces in the body, which is essential for optimal health in TCM.
- *Connecting to the Skin and Organ Systems:* According to TCM philosophy, the skin is a mirror of internal organ health. By treating the skin with Gua Sha, energy imbalances in deeper systems, like the liver or digestive system, can also be addressed.

5. **The Synergy of Science and Tradition:** Gua Sha bridges the gap between ancient wisdom and modern

science. While TCM highlights energy flow and holistic balance, contemporary research supports its physiological benefits:
- Studies show increased microcirculation after Gua Sha, with measurable reductions in muscle soreness and systemic inflammation.
- Observations indicate significant stimulation of the parasympathetic nervous system (responsible for relaxation), reinforcing its stress-relieving benefits.

By combining scientific validity with the intuitive understanding of the body's energy, Gua Sha presents a powerful method for improving overall health, healing, and skincare. Whether you practice it at home for self-care or seek professional treatments, this versatile practice continues to prove its enduring value.

The Gua Sha Tools

Gua Sha tools come in different materials, shapes, and designs, each suited for specific needs like facial rejuvenation or full-body massage. This chapter helps you choose the best tool to enhance your self-care routine.

Gua Sha Tools Based on Materials

The material of your Gua Sha tool plays a key role in how it feels, functions, and interacts with your skin. Let's take a closer look at some of the most popular materials available:

1. *Jade:* Jade, a staple in Traditional Chinese Medicine, is a popular choice for Gua Sha tools due to its cooling properties. It helps reduce puffiness and inflammation, while its smooth texture makes it perfect for gliding over delicate facial areas.
    - **Unique Properties:** Cool to the touch, even without refrigeration. Known for its durability and symbolic connection to balance and purity in TCM.
    - **Best Uses:** Facial treatments and neck massages.

- **Care Tips:** Given jade's porous nature, it should be cleaned thoroughly after each use to avoid bacterial build-up.
2. *Rose Quartz:* The soft pink hue of rose quartz is as soothing as the tool itself. Known as the "stone of love," rose quartz is thought to promote self-care and relaxation while improving circulation.
   - **Unique Properties:** Retains heat slightly better than jade, making it ideal for gentle, warming massages.
   - **Best Uses:** Facial Gua Sha for reducing redness and stress-induced puffiness.
   - **Care Tips:** Handle with care; rose quartz is more fragile than jade and can chip if dropped.
3. *Obsidian:* Obsidian, a volcanic glass, catches the eye with its striking black sheen. This material is thought to have grounding properties and is highly durable compared to more fragile stones like jade or rose quartz.
   - **Unique Properties:** Holds both heat and cold, providing versatility for soothing or energizing massages.
   - **Best Uses:** Targeting specific tension points on the neck, shoulders, or larger muscle groups.
   - **Care Tips:** Regular cleaning with soap and water will maintain obsidian's glass-like finish.

4. ***Amethyst:*** The deep purple hue of amethyst isn't just beautiful—it's also linked to healing and detoxifying properties. This crystal is believed to carry calming energies, making it perfect for stress relief.
    - **Unique Properties:** Smooth texture combined with supposed energy-clearing benefits.
    - **Best Uses:** Massage for stress-prone areas like the forehead, temples, and jawline.
    - **Care Tips:** Avoid exposure to harsh chemicals to ensure the tool retains its natural polish.
5. ***Bone or Horn:*** Bone and horn tools, often crafted from buffalo or ox horn, have been traditional Gua Sha tools for centuries. These are eco-friendly options favored in some practices due to their natural textures.
    - **Unique Properties:** Durable with a firmer pressure application, ideal for deep-tissue massage.
    - **Best Uses:** Body applications, especially for areas with tight muscles or tension.
    - **Care Tips:** Avoid soaking in water for extended periods, as this can weaken the material.
6. ***Plastic:*** Plastic Gua Sha tools are lightweight and budget-friendly, making them accessible for beginners. However, they don't carry the energetic properties associated with natural materials, and many people report a less luxurious feel.

- **Unique Properties:** Affordable and highly accessible.
- **Best Uses:** Beginners or experimental practice.
- **Care Tips:** Ensure the plastic is BPA-free and cleaned thoroughly after each use to prevent wear and tear.

Choosing the right Gua Sha tool depends on your needs, preferences, and the material's unique properties. Whether you prioritize tradition, durability, or affordability, there's a tool to enhance your self-care routine.

Gua Sha Tool Shapes and Their Applications

Along with the material, the shape of a Gua Sha tool determines where and how it can be used on the body. Each curvature and edge is designed for specific applications, ensuring precision in treatment.

1. *Standard Rectangular Shape:* This design features a flat body with rounded edges and is versatile for general use.
    - **Applications:** Ideal for both facial and body massage. Use on larger muscle groups like the legs, arms, and back.
    - **Best For:** Beginners or those looking for an all-purpose tool.

2. ***Heart Shape:*** Heart-shaped tools are widely loved for facial Gua Sha as they are tailored to fit the natural contours of the face.
    - **Applications:** Sculpting the jawline, lifting cheekbones, and working along the neck and forehead.
    - **Best For:** Those focusing on facial aesthetics and lymphatic drainage.
3. ***Spoon Shape:*** This spoon-like tool is ergonomically designed for larger areas, making it perfect for deep tissue Gua Sha work.
    - **Applications:** Relieving tension in the back, shoulders, and thighs.
    - **Best For:** Athletic recovery or deeper muscle relief.
4. ***Wing or Dolphin Shape:*** Inspired by the graceful curves of a dolphin or wing, this tool offers both pointed and rounded edges.
    - **Applications:** Precision work on the neck, around temples, or even the sides of the nose.
    - **Best For:** Sinus relief and releasing tension in smaller, delicate areas.
5. ***Chinese Coin Shape:*** Circular tools with raised ridges at the center mimic Chinese coins and are designed for stimulating larger muscle areas.
    - **Applications:** Treating areas like the back or thighs where deep pressure is required.

- **Best For:** Full-body massages aimed at circulation or muscular stiffness.

Choosing the right Gua Sha tool shape depends on your specific needs, whether it's facial sculpting, muscle relief, or full-body massage. With the proper tool, you can enhance your self-care routine and enjoy targeted, effective treatment.

How to Spot Authentic, High-Quality Gua Sha Tools

With the growing popularity of Gua Sha, the market has become saturated with counterfeit or low-quality tools. Keep these tips in mind when making your selection:

1. *Material Authenticity:* Check for genuine materials. Jade should feel cool to the touch and have visible natural variations, while plastic imitations often lack this quality.
2. *Weight and Texture:* Authentic tools will be weighty and smooth, not lightweight or slippery. A heavier tool often indicates a higher-quality material like real quartz or jade.
3. *Edge Finish:* The edges should feel smooth and polished without any sharp or rough areas. Poorly finished tools can irritate or even damage your skin.
4. *Reputable Sellers:* Purchase from trusted stores or online platforms specializing in skincare and wellness.

Look for certifications or positive customer reviews to ensure quality.
5. ***Price Point:*** While price isn't always an indicator of quality, extremely cheap tools are often made from synthetic or low-quality materials. Invest in a tool that balances affordability with craftsmanship—your skin will thank you.
6. ***Packaging and Branding:*** High-quality tools often come with detailed instructions, a care pouch, or branded packaging. Be cautious of products that lack these details.
7. ***Test for Real Jade or Quartz:*** Real stone will not easily scratch or chip, so a quick test is to scratch the surface lightly with a key. Counterfeit versions often show signs of wear.

Choosing the right Gua Sha tool depends on your goals. For reducing puffiness and sculpting, try a heart-shaped rose quartz tool. For deeper pressure on sore muscles, opt for a wing-shaped obsidian tool. Beginners can start with a rectangular jade tool for versatility. Focus on material, shape, and craftsmanship to find a high-quality tool that enhances your Gua Sha practice.

How do Practitioners Perform the Gua Sha Technique?

The practice of gua sha, which is a kind of traditional Chinese medicine, consists of scraping the surface of the skin with a smooth, flat item. Gua sha is used to break up congestion and stagnation in the body, which enables the body to heal itself. This is the objective of the practice. The treatment of colds, the flu, and other respiratory conditions frequently involve the use of gua sha.

Any object that is smooth and flat can be used to make gua sha; however, the typical tool for the technique is a soup spoon or coin made of ceramic. The therapist will massage the client's skin using this instrument. This causes the formation of petechiae, which are very small dots that might be red, purple, or blue. These marks are an indication that the treatment is having the desired effect.

The massage therapist will start by applying lotion or oil to the client's skin. They will then use a smooth-edged tool, like a coin, to gently massage the skin in one direction, applying a reasonable amount of pressure. Strokes are continued until the skin turns red or "sha" (petechiae) develops, indicating the therapy's effectiveness by releasing stagnation in the body.

After a gua sha treatment, the therapist massages leftover oil into the skin and may apply heat for comfort. While the process is usually painless, some may experience mild stinging that fades quickly. Gua sha is safe and effective but should be avoided on painful areas.

How Often Should Gua Sha be Performed?

The goal of gua sha is to improve circulation while also breaking up congestion in the body. It is frequently utilized as a treatment for the common cold, influenza, and sinus infections. Many people feel that gua sha may boost both their energy levels and their general well-being.

For optimal effects, Gua Sha should be practiced twice and thrice each week. When treating acute disorders, it can be done daily. If you are new to Gua Sha, you should begin by performing the technique once or twice a week and gradually build up to the whole session. Always pay attention to what your body is telling you, and put your faith in your instincts.

Gua Sha can be practiced on any part of the body where there is congestion or obstruction, including the face, the neck, the chest, the back, and anyplace else on the body. It is important to steer clear of any regions of damaged skin, open sores, rashes, or inflammation. Before doing Gua Sha on yourself or anyone else, you should seek the advice of a trained practitioner if you have any questions.

Gua Sha is a simple and effective healing method that can be practiced at home with minimal tools. Regular practice can improve circulation, relieve congestion and cold symptoms, and boost energy levels. Always listen to your body and trust your instincts. If you're new to Gua Sha, start slowly and build up gradually. For questions or concerns, consult a skilled practitioner.

Uses of Gua Sha

It is believed that by promoting the flow of blood and lymph, gua sha can enhance circulation and speed up the healing process. Gua sha is utilized for the treatment of pain the vast majority of the time; however, it may also be utilized for the treatment of other ailments such as the common cold, headaches, and digestive difficulties.

Although there is not a lot of data to back up the claims that are made about gua sha, a few studies have suggested that the procedure can assist to alleviate pain and inflammation.

Here are some of the uses of gua sha:

Treating Pain and Inflammation

According to traditional Chinese medicine, the Gua Sha method can help break up stagnation and promote circulation. Gua sha is frequently utilized as a treatment for a variety of diseases, including pain and inflammation. Inflammatory disorders including arthritis, carpal tunnel syndrome, fibromyalgia, and tendonitis are expected to benefit particularly well from exercise since it is supposed to reduce pain and improve mobility.

Boosting Immunity

It is believed that gua sha can improve immune function by accelerating lymphatic drainage. Lymph is a transparent fluid that plays a role in the elimination of waste and poisons from the body. It is believed that the technique can aid in the treatment of several diseases, including the common cold and the flu.

Relieving Stress

It is believed that by increasing circulation and encouraging the body's natural production of endorphins, gua sha can help relieve tension and promote relaxation. In the treatment of illnesses such as anxiety, headaches, and sleeplessness, gua sha is frequently utilized as a supplemental therapy.

There has only been a little amount of study done in a scientific setting to determine whether or not Gua Sha is effective; nonetheless, many who have tried it claim that it helps them feel calmer and less anxious after a session.

Relieving Fatigue

It is believed that gua sha can help reduce fatigue by improving circulation and assisting the body in eliminating toxins from the system. It is believed that engaging in this activity can assist in the treatment of diseases such as chronic fatigue syndrome and fibromyalgia.

Relieving Headaches

Gua sha is believed to help relieve headaches by improving blood circulation and easing muscle tension, which can be common triggers for head pain. By gently scraping the skin with a gua sha tool, the practice may reduce inflammation and promote relaxation, making it a potential remedy for migraines and tension headaches. Many people report feeling a soothing release of pressure, which can bring comfort and relief from persistent discomfort.

Improving Digestion

It is believed that the practice of gua sha might enhance digestion by enhancing the movement of blood and lymph. It is believed that the technique might assist ease blockages in the digestive system and break up stagnation in the body.

People who suffer from indigestion, bloating, and constipation are claimed to benefit from the technique since it helps relieve those symptoms. Even though there is no proof from scientific studies to back up these claims, a lot of individuals feel that using gua sha can be an efficient technique to enhance digestion.

Treating Flu

It is believed that gua sha can strengthen the immune system, increase the movement of lymph, and decrease inflammation. There is a school of thought that holds that gua sha can be used to treat influenza by alleviating the symptoms of the illness and assisting the body in fighting off the virus.

Gua sha is a harmless and mild therapy that may bring some comfort to patients who are suffering from the flu, even though there is no scientific proof to support the claims being made about its efficacy.

Detoxifying the Body

It is believed that the gua sha technique might assist in the detoxification process of the body by increasing the circulation of blood and lymph.

Acne, eczema, and psoriasis are just some of the skin diseases that are said to respond well to treatment with gua sha. Those who subscribe to this school of thought hold the belief that scraping can aid in the elimination of toxins from the body and boost circulation.

Relieving Menstrual Cramps

It is said that gua sha is particularly useful for alleviating the cramping associated with menstruation. Many women report that they suffer from pain and discomfort during their periods because of impaired circulation.

It is believed that the strokes of gua sha might enhance blood flow, which in turn reduces inflammation and provides relief from cramps. In addition, it is believed that engaging in the practice can assist in the regulation of hormones and lower levels of stress, both of which are factors that might contribute to menstruation discomfort.

For Skincare

It is believed that gua sha can improve circulation and assist the skin in more effectively absorbing skincare products. It is common practice to utilize gua sha in combination with face massage because of the widespread belief that doing so confers several health advantages. A more youthful look is one of the benefits, along with an enhanced skin tone and a reduction in puffiness.

As a cosmetic therapy, gua sha is gaining more and more attention these days, and many professionals in the field of skincare feel that it has the potential to completely disrupt the business.

Gua sha is a therapy that is both safe and delicate, and it may be utilized to bring about the alleviation of a wide variety of illnesses. It is believed that gua sha may strengthen the immune system, reduce stress, enhance digestion, treat influenza, cleanse the body, alleviate menstruation cramps, and improve skin care.

While there is minimal scientific evidence to support these claims, many people who have tried gua sha report feeling calmer and having less stress following a session. This is even though there is limited scientific evidence to support these claims. People who are suffering from a range of diseases may find some relief from their symptoms via the use of the safe and gentle treatment known as gua sha.

For the Body

Beyond skincare, gua sha can provide profound relief and benefits when applied to the body. From alleviating muscle tension to improving circulation, body gua sha targets specific areas with effective results. Here's how you can use it to address common concerns.

Relieving Neck, Shoulders, and Back Pain

If you suffer from tight, sore neck muscles or back pain from stress or poor posture, gua sha can offer relief by releasing muscle tension, improving flexibility, and enhancing circulation.

Neck Pain:

1. Apply a layer of oil to your neck to ensure smooth strokes.
2. Hold the gua sha tool at an angle and start at the base of your neck.

3. Use upward strokes, moving towards your hairline using light to medium pressure.
4. Glide the tool downward from the jawline to the collarbone if you want to encourage lymphatic drainage.
5. Repeat each stroke 5-7 times, focusing on tense areas.

Shoulder Pain:

1. Massage oil over your shoulders to prevent skin irritation.
2. With the curved edge of the gua sha tool, glide outward from the base of your neck toward your shoulder.
3. Use medium pressure for 5-8 firm strokes on each side.
4. Pay attention to areas where stiffness or knots are concentrated.

Back Pain: (Ideal with the assistance of a partner)

1. Apply oil along both sides of the spine. Avoid scraping directly on the bones.
2. With a flat-edged gua sha tool, glide it upward from the lower back toward the shoulders using firm, even strokes.
3. Focus on one side of the back at a time. Repeat each stroke 5-7 times.

4. Use slower motions for tight or knotty areas to release deep tension.

Pro Tip: Loosen muscles with a warm bath or hot compress before your session to increase comfort and efficacy.

Improving Circulation and Reducing Cellulite in Legs

Gua sha can also enhance circulation in the legs, relieving heaviness, promoting lymph flow, and potentially reducing cellulite. With regular practice, these techniques can leave your legs feeling rejuvenated.

Steps:

1. Apply oil or body lotion liberally over your thighs and calves.
2. Use a flat-edged or comb-shaped gua sha tool.
3. For the thighs, glide the tool from the knees upward toward the hips. Use firm, steady strokes and repeat 6-8 times on each area.
4. For the calves, begin at the ankles and sweep upward toward the knees. Use medium pressure.
5. On cellulite-prone areas, apply firmer strokes with a focus on consistency and smoothness.

Suggestion: Incorporate these sessions 3-5 times per week and stay hydrated afterward for optimal results.

Resolving Common Issues

Gua sha is also excellent for managing localized issues such as carpal tunnel syndrome or tight calves resulting from repetitive strain or physical activity.

Relieving Carpal Tunnel Syndrome:

1. Gently massage oil onto your wrists and forearms.
2. Use a smaller gua sha tool and glide from your wrist toward your forearm in straight, consistent strokes. Repeat 5-8 times.
3. Finish by gliding the tool outward from the palm of your hand towards each finger.

Easing Tight Calves:

1. Apply oil for smoother gliding.
2. Start at the Achilles tendon (above the heel) and move the tool upward toward the back of the knee in smooth strokes.
3. Use medium pressure and repeat the motion 8-10 times per calf.
4. Pause and lightly circle around knots or sore spots to release tightness.

Pro Tip: Follow up with gentle stretching for enhanced benefits and relaxation.

By incorporating these gua sha techniques into your self-care routine, you can extend its benefits across your entire body.

Whether you're looking to relieve pain, improve blood flow, or just feel more relaxed, this ancient practice has a place in holistic wellness. Regular use not only provides physical comfort but also encourages a deeper connection to your body, making gua sha a valuable tool for modern self-care.

Gua Sha for Specific Health Conditions

Gua sha is an ancient healing practice that offers natural relief for various health conditions. Beyond relaxation, it uses simple, intentional strokes to address discomfort like headaches, muscle pain, or even digestive issues. This chapter outlines easy-to-follow techniques to manage some of the most common ailments using gua sha.

Alleviating Tension Headaches and Migraines

Headaches and migraines can disrupt your day, often caused by stress, muscle tension, or poor circulation. Gua sha focuses on relaxing tight muscles and improving blood flow, offering a soothing remedy for this discomfort.

Steps to Relieve Headaches:
1. Begin by applying a thin layer of oil to your forehead, temples, and neck for smooth strokes.
2. Use a flat gua sha tool and gently glide outward from the center of your forehead toward your temples.

Apply light pressure and repeat this 6-8 times for each side.
3. Gently scrape along your hairline, starting from the middle of your forehead and moving toward your ears. This stroke can help release tension.
4. Work on your temples using small, circular motions with the edge or corner of the tool. Massage for about 30 seconds to 1 minute on each side.
5. Lastly, relieve tight neck muscles by gliding the tool upward from the base of your neck to the base of your skull. Use medium pressure and repeat 5-7 times.

Bonus Tip: Create a calming space while performing this routine—dim lighting and deep breaths can enhance its relaxing effects.

Managing Arthritis and Fibromyalgia Symptoms

Both arthritis and fibromyalgia may cause chronic stiffness, inflammation, and overall discomfort. Gua sha can work as a gentle tool to promote blood circulation, ease tension, and provide relief in inflamed or painful areas.

Steps for Arthritis Relief:
1. Target the painful or stiff joint and add a light layer of oil for smooth strokes.

2. Use a small gua sha tool to glide in circular, sweeping motions around the affected joint. Be gentle and repeat 8-10 times.
3. If the area feels swollen, focus on gentle outward strokes, moving away from the joint toward major lymph nodes like those under your arm or behind your knees. This can help reduce puffiness.

Fibromyalgia Support:
1. For muscle aches in areas like the shoulders, thighs, or back, start with oil application to the affected regions.
2. Perform long, slow strokes with the flat side of the gua sha tool along the muscle groups. Repetition of 6-8 times per area is ideal.
3. Avoid pressing too hard on tender spots—instead, use lighter pressure for a soothing effect. Circular motions can help on extra-sensitive areas.

<u>**Note:**</u> Always listen to your body's limits. Avoid applying too much pressure or working too long over delicate areas.

Easing Menstrual Cramps

Menstrual cramps can range from mild to incapacitating, often caused by muscle tension and inflammation in the lower abdomen. Gua sha may help soothe pain and reduce cramping when used gently around the abdominal area.

Steps to Relieve Cramps:

1. Lie down in a comfortable position and apply a warming oil or lotion to your abdomen.
2. With your gua sha tool, use small circular motions around your navel for 1-2 minutes to stimulate circulation.
3. Move the tool in horizontal strokes across your lower abdomen, just below your belly button. Repeat this motion 8-10 times with gentle pressure.
4. Go for long, slow strokes on each side of your abdomen, moving from the navel toward your hips.

Pro Tip: Pair your gua sha session with a warm compress or herbal tea to further calm the cramps and relax your body.

Promoting Digestion

Digestive problems like bloating or constipation often result from stress, sluggish circulation, or blocked energy in the abdominal area. Gua sha can help stimulate lymph flow and digestive organs, making it a useful option for supporting gut health.

Steps for Better Digestion:

1. Apply oil to your abdominal area, ensuring even coverage.

2. Begin with downward strokes from your ribcage toward your lower belly. Use consistent motions and repeat 6-8 times.
3. Perform circular, clockwise strokes around your belly button, mimicking the natural movement of digestion. Do this for 1-2 minutes.
4. For bloating or discomfort on the sides of your stomach, gently glide the tool from your lower ribs down toward your hips using medium pressure.

Tip: Practicing gua sha after meals or when you feel bloated can help ease discomfort and promote smoother digestion.

Gua sha offers a natural, non-invasive way to handle health concerns. With these targeted techniques, you can alleviate headaches, manage chronic pain, and support your body's overall wellness.

Regular practice allows you to take charge of your health, making gua sha a valuable addition to your self-care routine. Whether you're addressing physical discomfort or seeking a moment of relaxation, gua sha is a versatile companion in achieving balance and relief.

How Gua Sha Treatment Complements Other Traditional Chinese Medicine (TCM) Practices

Traditional Chinese Medicine (TCM) has been a key part of Chinese culture for centuries. Built on the idea of achieving balance and harmony within the body, its practices focus on unblocking the flow of energy, or Qi, through a network of channels called meridians. Among the many therapeutic techniques used in TCM is Gua Sha, a treatment that involves using a smooth tool to scrape the skin, stimulating circulation and relieving tension.

While Gua Sha is a powerful therapy in its own right, its true strength shines when used alongside other TCM practices like acupuncture, Chinese herbal medicine, cupping, and massage. Together, these approaches create a holistic synergy that enhances the body's natural healing process.

How Gua Sha Complements TCM Techniques

1. Gua Sha and Acupuncture

Acupuncture and Gua Sha are key practices in TCM, working together to clear energy blockages and restore balance. Acupuncture uses needles on specific meridian points to stimulate Qi, while Gua Sha involves scraping strokes to release tension across larger areas.

Together, they can deliver powerful results. For example, a patient with chronic neck pain might receive acupuncture to reduce inflammation and calm nerves, followed by Gua Sha on the shoulders and upper back to loosen muscles and boost circulation. This combination often speeds up recovery and provides lasting pain relief.

2. Gua Sha and Chinese Herbal Medicine

Chinese herbal medicine complements TCM's external treatments by addressing imbalances at their root. Herbal remedies often target issues like stress, pain, or immune support. Paired with Gua Sha, they create a balanced internal and external approach.

For instance, Gua Sha boosts blood flow and aids toxin release, enhancing the effects of detoxifying herbs. Similarly, anti-inflammatory herbs prepare the body for therapies like Gua Sha, working together for a more complete healing experience.

3. Gua Sha and Cupping

Gua Sha and cupping share some similarities—they both promote healthy blood circulation and draw out stagnant energy. However, their mechanisms differ. Cupping uses suction to pull stagnant blood, toxins, and Qi to the surface of the skin, while Gua Sha uses stroking to move these blockages through the channels.

How do these two practices complement each other? A practitioner may start with cupping to draw out deeper blockages in the muscles and meridians, then follow with Gua Sha to smooth the flow of energy and encourage the body to process those released blockages.

4. Gua Sha and Massage

Massage therapy is another ancient technique that pairs beautifully with Gua Sha. While massage focuses on kneading and pressing muscles to relieve tension, Gua Sha works on stimulating the underlying energy pathways and improving circulation. Together, they address both the physical and energetic aspects of an ailment.

A common application involves treating someone experiencing stress-induced shoulder and neck tightness. Massage can help relax the musculoskeletal system and release emotional tension, while Gua Sha further enhances blood and Qi movement across the same areas. The result is a deeply relaxing and therapeutic experience that targets the root of the tension.

The Role of Meridians and Energy Flow in Gua Sha Therapy

At the core of TCM lies the concept of meridians, a network of invisible pathways through which Qi flows. Blockages, stagnation, or imbalances in these pathways are believed to result in illness, pain, or emotional disturbances. Gua Sha's stroking techniques work to address these disruptions by stimulating the surface layers of the skin, encouraging both Qi and blood to flow freely.

When applied to specific meridians, Gua Sha can target key organs and systems in the body. For example, scraping along the lung meridian helps detoxify the respiratory system, while stimulating the stomach meridian can aid digestion. By unblocking these energy highways, Gua Sha supports the body in achieving its natural state of harmony.

Case studies from TCM practitioners using Gua Sha in treatments.

1. **Chronic Neck Pain Relief**

   A randomized controlled trial demonstrated that Gua Sha significantly reduced neck pain severity and improved functional status in patients with chronic mechanical neck pain. The study also noted improvements in quality of life after just one treatment session.

   Read the study here:

   https://bit.ly/ChronicNeckPainRelief.

2. **Shoulder Pain and Restless Leg Syndrome (RLS)**

   This case study explored the use of Gua Sha to treat chronic shoulder pain, which unexpectedly led to improvements in the patient's restless leg syndrome. The treatment involved four sessions, resulting in reduced pain and better sleep quality.

   Read the study here:

   https://bit.ly/ShoulderPainRLS.

3. **Hepatoprotection in Chronic Hepatitis B**

   A case study showed that Gua Sha reduced liver inflammation markers (ALT and AST) in a patient with chronic active hepatitis B. The treatment also increased heme oxygenase-1 (HO-1), which has anti-inflammatory and hepatoprotective effects.

Read the study here:

https://bit.ly/HepatoChroHepaB.

4. **Improved Microcirculation and Pain Relief**

   This study highlighted Gua Sha's ability to enhance blood flow and reduce pain in chronic back and neck conditions. It discussed the neurobiological mechanisms, including stimulation of peripheral nociceptors and spinal cord pathways.

   Read the study here:

   https://bit.ly/MicrocirculationPR.

These case studies provide a glimpse into the practical applications of Gua Sha in Traditional Chinese Medicine, showcasing its versatility in addressing various health conditions.

Gua Sha is a powerful treatment that becomes even more effective when combined with other TCM practices like cupping, acupuncture, and herbal remedies. This holistic approach addresses both symptoms and root causes, promoting lasting relief and improved vitality by treating the mind, body, and spirit as one.

The Risks of the Gua Sha Technique

Gua Sha is generally considered a safe and effective practice when performed by a trained professional. However, it's important to be aware of potential risks or side effects to ensure a safe experience. Below are some common risks and how to avoid them:

1. ***Skin Bruising:*** Bruising is a common side effect of Gua Sha, varying based on skin sensitivity and pressure. These marks are typically harmless and fade within days, but it's important to avoid applying too much force.
2. ***Petechiae:*** Gua Sha can cause petechiae—small red or purple spots on the skin due to broken blood vessels. This is a natural response and typically clears up on its own within a few days.
3. ***Skin Infection:*** Using Gua Sha on open wounds or unclean skin can increase the risk of infection due to bacteria.

How to Avoid These Risks:

- *Use Clean Tools:* Always ensure tools are sterilized before treatment.
- *Prepare the Skin:* Cleanse the skin thoroughly before starting to remove any dirt or bacteria.
- *Avoid Damaged Skin:* Refrain from performing Gua Sha on areas with open cuts, wounds, or active infections.
- *Communicate:* Inform your practitioner of any injuries or sensitive areas to prevent unnecessary irritation.

Gua Sha can significantly improve circulation and ease pain when done correctly. To ensure safety, consult a knowledgeable practitioner or healthcare provider if you have any concerns about its suitability based on your skin or health condition.

Common Mistakes and How to Avoid Them

Gua Sha is an effective healing technique, but proper technique is essential. Avoiding common mistakes ensures a safe and beneficial practice. Here's a quick guide to help you perfect your Gua Sha experience.

1. **Misusing the Tools**

   Mistake: Using tools incorrectly or choosing the wrong shape for the area you're working on. Some beginners also use sharp objects or tools not designed for Gua Sha, which can hurt your skin.

How to Avoid It: Choose a quality Gua Sha tool made of jade, rose quartz, or stainless steel, selecting shapes suited for specific areas. Use gentle, one-directional strokes for the best results.

2. **Applying Too Much Pressure**

   Mistake: Pressing too hard can cause pain or leave excessive bruising, which isn't necessary for Gua Sha to work.

   How to Avoid It: Start with light to moderate pressure to stimulate blood flow without causing pain. Gradually increase pressure if needed, but avoid going too hard initially.

3. **Skipping Essential Steps**

   Mistake: Forgetting to apply oil or prep your skin. Dry "scraping" can cause irritation and discomfort.

   How to Avoid It: Cleanse your skin, apply facial oil or lotion, and gently massage to prepare for smooth and effective tool use.

4. **Over-Scraping**

   Mistake: Spending too much time on one area or doing multiple sessions in one day. Over-scraping can lead to irritation, excessive bruising, and even damage your skin.

How to Avoid It: Limit sessions to 10-15 minutes per area and take breaks. Stop if redness or small red spots appear, as it indicates over-stimulation.

5. **Ignoring Contraindications**

   Mistake: Using Gua Sha in areas where it's not safe, such as on open wounds, thin or fragile skin, or over varicose veins. Some people also use Gua Sha without considering their health conditions, which might make it unsafe.

   How to Avoid It: Avoid Gua Sha if you have skin issues, bruise easily, or are pregnant without consulting a healthcare provider. Prioritize safety!

Final Tips for a Better Gua Sha Experience

- *Stay consistent, not aggressive:* A few gentle sessions over time are more effective than one harsh session.
- *Listen to your body:* Pay attention to how your skin reacts and adjust your technique accordingly.
- *Hydrate:* Drink water before and after Gua Sha to help flush out toxins and keep your body refreshed.

By avoiding these common pitfalls, you'll see the amazing benefits Gua Sha has to offer—without the discomfort or unwanted side effects.

Gua Sha Safety Tips: Practicing Safely and Effectively

Gua Sha is a powerful and relaxing wellness practice with many benefits. However, to make the most of it, you need to focus on safety and proper use. Neglecting these guidelines can lead to discomfort or even harm. Here's everything you need to know about practicing Gua Sha safely and effectively!

When to Avoid Gua Sha

While Gua Sha is a versatile technique, there are situations where it might not be the best choice. Knowing when to skip it is essential to protect your health:

- *If You're Pregnant:* Gua Sha can be stimulating and may not be suitable during pregnancy, especially on the abdomen or lower back. Always consult a healthcare provider before proceeding.
- *On Open Wounds or Irritated Skin:* Avoid using Gua Sha over cuts, scrapes, burns, rashes, or sensitive areas to prevent pain and infection.
- *If You're on Blood Thinners:* Gua Sha increases blood flow, and if you're taking blood-thinning medication or have a bleeding disorder, it could cause excessive bruising.
- *Fragile Skin or Health Conditions:* Be cautious if you have fragile, thin skin or underlying conditions like

varicose veins or active infections. A gentle approach is key.

When in doubt, consult with a healthcare professional or TCM practitioner to determine if Gua Sha is safe for you.

Recognizing Signs of Overuse or Improper Technique

Using Gua Sha correctly is vital for an effective and pain-free experience. Watch for these red flags that might indicate overuse or incorrect methods:

- *Excessive Redness or Bruising:* Mild redness and slight petechiae are normal, but if your skin becomes very bruised, swollen, or painful, it could mean you're pressing too hard or using the tool for too long.
- *Lingering Discomfort:* Gua Sha should feel therapeutic, not painful. If soreness lasts beyond a day or two, it's a sign to lighten your pressure or reduce session frequency.
- *Uneven or Erratic Strokes:* Strokes that are too fast, uneven, or back-and-forth can irritate the skin. Stick to slow, consistent movements in one direction for the best results.

Remember, with Gua Sha, less is often more. Gentle, mindful techniques go a long way in achieving its benefits.

Maintaining Hygiene and Cleaning Tools

Cleanliness is a crucial part of practicing Gua Sha, as your tools are in direct contact with your skin. Dirty tools can lead to irritation or infection, so here's how to keep them clean and safe:

1. ***Wash Your Tools After Each Use:*** Use warm water and gentle soap to clean your Gua Sha tool thoroughly. Rinse well and dry with a clean towel.
2. ***Sanitize Regularly:*** For extra safety, sanitize your tool using rubbing alcohol or an antibacterial wipe. This is especially important if you're using it on more than one person.
3. ***Store Properly:*** Keep your tools in a clean, dry place, like a pouch or case, to protect them from dust and bacteria.
4. ***Start with Clean Skin and Hands:*** Wash your hands and face (or area being treated) before each session to create a hygienic environment for Gua Sha.

By following these steps, you'll ensure a clean and safe Gua Sha experience every time.

Final Tips for Safe Gua Sha Practice

- ***Listen to Your Body:*** Pay attention to how your skin and muscles respond. If something feels off, adjust your pressure or technique.

- ***Use Quality Tools and Products:*** Choose Gua Sha tools made of materials like jade, rose quartz, or stainless steel, and pair them with a safe facial or body oil to reduce friction.
- ***Hydrate and Rest:*** Drinking water after a session helps flush out toxins, while allowing your body time to recover ensures the best results.

By keeping these safety guidelines in mind, you'll be able to unlock the full benefits of Gua Sha while keeping your body protected and happy.

Is Gua Sha Right for Me?

When conducted appropriately by a trained practitioner, gua sha is usually regarded as safe for most individuals; however, specific precautions should be taken if you have certain ailments or health concerns. Before you use gua sha, you should be sure to get advice from a qualified medical practitioner if you have any of the following conditions:

1. ***Bleeding Disorders:*** Gua sha should not be performed on people with bleeding disorders or low platelet counts, as the process can cause bruising and bleeding.
2. ***Open Wounds:*** If you have any open cuts or scrapes on your skin, it is important to avoid gua sha until they have healed. Otherwise, you run the risk of infection.
3. ***Fragile Skin:*** If you have sensitive or fragile skin, it is important to be extra careful when performing gua sha.

Be sure to use a very light touch and avoid any areas that are inflamed or irritated. If you experience any pain or discomfort, discontinue the treatment immediately.
4. ***Circulatory Problems:*** If you have any circulatory problems, it is important to consult with a healthcare professional before trying gua sha. The process can cause dizziness in some people, so it is important to be aware of this before starting the treatment.
5. ***Heart Conditions:*** Gua sha should not be performed on people with heart conditions, as the process can cause an increase in heart rate.
6. ***Pregnant or Breastfeeding:*** If you are pregnant or breastfeeding, it is important to consult with a healthcare professional before trying gua sha. There is not enough research on the effects of gua sha during pregnancy and breastfeeding, so it is best to err on the side of caution.
7. ***Those Who are Taking Blood Thinners:*** If you are taking blood thinners, it is important to consult with a healthcare professional before trying gua sha. The process can cause bruising and bleeding, so it is important to be aware of this before starting the treatment.

Overall, gua sha can be a great way to improve circulation and promote relaxation; however, it is important to consult with a healthcare professional before trying this treatment if you have any underlying health conditions or concerns.

Women and Facial Beauty

It is challenging to be a woman and to refrain from continually comparing oneself to other women. In particular about the attractiveness of the face. We are the harshest judges of ourselves, and it appears that no matter what we try, we will never be able to live up to the expectations that we have for ourselves.

It seems like there is an endless list of things to improve about one's appearance, whether it be getting rid of dark circles or finally attaining that dewy sheen. Let's take a look at some of the many different face battles that women have to fight.

Acne is one of the most widespread face problems that women experience throughout their lifetimes. Several different variables can lead to acne, including hormones, heredity, and even stress. Even though there are several different over-the-counter remedies, there are instances when they just aren't enough.

In severe circumstances, you might even need to consult a dermatologist about the condition. Wrinkles are a problem that many people have with their faces. A decrease in the amount of collagen and elastin in the skin is what leads to wrinkles. This can be caused by a variety of factors, including aging, sun damage, smoking, etc.

Uneven skin tone is another typical facial concern that a majority of women have to deal with. This could be the result of several factors, including prolonged exposure to the sun, melasma, or post-inflammatory hyperpigmentation. Last but not least, we have bags under our eyes. Several factors can lead to dark circles around the eyes, including being dehydrated, not getting enough sleep, having allergies, and so on.

Throughout the years, a variety of potential remedies to assist women with their face issues have been presented. Some of these answers are grounded in cultural ideas, while others are grounded in research conducted in scientific fields. Even while no cure is certain to work for every woman, some therapies are successful for the vast majority of women.

Benefits of Using Gua Sha on your Face

Women have been utilizing facial treatments for several years to improve their complexion and overall look. Women have utilized a wide variety of methods, dating back to ancient Egypt and continuing right up until the present day in Hollywood, in their pursuit of a more youthful appearance.

Today, the Western world is beginning to understand the benefits of gua sha for skin care, and the method is growing in popularity as a means to create a young appearance.

1. *Reduce the appearance of wrinkles:* Gua sha is popular for reducing wrinkles and fine lines, with some anecdotal evidence suggesting it may boost collagen production and improve skin appearance, though more research is needed.
2. *Improves skin tone and texture:* Gua sha technique stimulates circulation and promotes lymph drainage, which can improve skin tone, and texture and promote a healthy glow.

3. ***Release muscle tension and toxins:*** The massage technique helps to release muscle tension and toxins that can build up in the skin, giving you a healthier and more youthful appearance.
4. ***Reduce puffiness:*** When performed on the face, gua sha can help to reduce puffiness and promote circulation. It can also help to drain lymphatic fluid, which can reduce the appearance of under-eye bags.
5. ***Reduce puffiness and inflammation:*** Gua sha is a traditional Chinese medicine practice that involves scraping the face with a smooth tool to reduce puffiness and inflammation. It's believed to boost circulation, promote drainage, and leave skin looking brighter and more radiant.
6. ***Helps improve the absorption of skincare products:*** Additionally, gua sha can help improve the absorption of skincare products. The massage technique helps to open up the pores and allow the product to penetrate deeper into the skin.
7. ***Sculpt the face:*** Gua sha can also be used to sculpt the face, contouring the jawline and cheekbones. When performed correctly, Gua sha can give the face a lift and help to improve its overall appearance.
8. ***Release sinus pressure:*** Gua sha is often used on the face, and it is said to help reduce sinus pressure and relieve pain. Gua sha is thought to work by stimulating the flow of Qi, or life energy, in the body. This

increased circulation is said to promote healing and ease pain and congestion.

Many women are now using gua sha as part of their regular beauty routine. Gua sha can be done at home or a spa. If you're looking for a way to achieve a youthful appearance, gua sha may be worth trying. The skincare benefits of gua sha are now being recognized by the Western world, and the technique is becoming increasingly popular as a way to achieve a youthful appearance.

Facial Gua Sha for Targeted Concerns

Facial gua sha isn't just a relaxing practice—it can also address specific issues like puffiness, wrinkles, and sinus discomfort. With the right techniques, you can target these concerns in your routine. Here's how to tailor gua sha to meet your specific needs:

Reducing Under-Eye Puffiness and Dark Circles

The skin under your eyes is delicate, so light, gentle strokes are key in this area. Gua sha can help reduce puffiness by improving circulation and moving trapped fluids.

Steps:

1. Apply a hydrating eye cream or facial oil around the eye area for smooth gliding.
2. Using the smallest, curved edge of your gua sha tool, start at the inner corner of your eye.

3. Gently glide the tool outward toward your temple, following the natural curve of your eye socket. Keep the pressure very light.
4. Repeat this motion 3-5 times per side.

Tip: For extra soothing, place your gua sha tool in the fridge before use. The cool touch can help reduce swelling faster.

Sculpting the Jawline and Cheekbones

Facial gua sha can help contour and define the jawline and cheekbones by boosting circulation and releasing tightness in those areas.

Steps for the Jawline:
1. Start at the center of your chin and apply a little facial oil along your jawline.
2. Use the curved edge of the tool and glide it from the chin outward toward your ear.
3. Apply medium pressure and make slow, steady strokes.
4. Repeat 5-10 times on each side.

Steps for the Cheekbones:
1. Place the tool beside your nose, using the curved edge.
2. Slowly glide it upwards along your cheekbone toward your temple.
3. Use medium pressure but be gentle enough to avoid discomfort.

4. Repeat 5-8 times on each side.

Pro Tip: Lift the skin by moving in upward motions rather than dragging downward.

Minimizing Fine Lines and Wrinkles

Facial gua sha can reduce the appearance of fine lines by increasing blood flow and gently massaging tight muscles beneath the skin. Regular practice can soften lines on the forehead, around the mouth, and in other common areas.

Steps:

1. Apply a nourishing, anti-aging serum to the targeted areas.
2. For the forehead, hold the tool flat and glide upwards from your brows to your hairline.
3. For laugh lines, start at the side of your nose and glide the tool outward to the cheeks.
4. Use light to medium pressure and repeat each motion 5-8 times.

Reminder: Gua sha doesn't erase wrinkles, but it can make your skin appear smoother and more refreshed over time.

Performing Gua Sha for Sinus Relief

Gua sha is great for easing sinus congestion and discomfort, especially during allergy season or colds. The process encourages lymphatic drainage and reduces pressure around your nose and eyebrows.

Steps:

1. Apply a facial oil to the center of your face.
2. Use the tool's flat edge and glide it from the sides of your nose outward toward your ears.
3. For your eyebrows, glide the tool gently across your brow bone, moving from the center of your forehead toward the temples.
4. Use light to medium pressure, repeating each movement 5-6 times.

Tip: Breathing deeply while performing these strokes can enhance relaxation and help you feel less stuffy.

Stress Reduction with Gua Sha

Facial gua sha is not only great for physical benefits but also for calming the mind. By massaging areas prone to tension, you can reduce stress and promote relaxation.

Steps:

1. Use a flat, smooth tool and apply oil to your temples.
2. Glide the tool in slow, circular strokes around your temples and forehead.

3. For the jaw, glide the tool upward from the chin toward the ears to release tension held in the jaw muscles.
4. Repeat each motion for about 1-2 minutes, focusing on areas that feel tight.

Bonus Tip: Dim the lights or play relaxing music during your session to deepen the calming effects.

Facial gua sha is versatile and easy to customize to meet your skin's needs. Whether you're looking to reduce puffiness, soften wrinkles, or just relax after a busy day, these simple techniques can help you feel and look your best. With practice, these movements will become second nature, making gua sha a perfect addition to your self-care routine.

5 Step-by-Step Guide on How to Perform Gua Sha

Gua Sha is an age-old practice that offers numerous skincare benefits, such as reducing fine lines, improving skin tone, and relieving facial tension. While it may seem intimidating for beginners, this guide will break it down into simple steps that you can easily follow at home to achieve radiant, youthful skin.

Step 1: Choose the Right Gua Sha Tool for Your Needs

The first step to successful Gua Sha is selecting the right tool tailored for specific areas or purposes. Gua Sha tools come in a variety of shapes and materials, and each serves unique functions:

- *For the Face and Neck:* A heart-shaped or S-shaped Gua Sha tool works best for the face, fitting the natural contours, such as the jawline or cheekbones. These tools are gentle and effective for intricate, smaller areas.

- ***For the Body:*** Flat, wider tools are ideal for broader areas like the back, shoulders, or legs as they cover more surface area and can handle more pressure.
- ***For the Undereye Area:*** Use a slender, smooth, and flat-edged tool. The material is equally important—opt for cooling stones like jade or rose quartz for the delicate under-eye area.

Tip for Beginners: Go for tools made of materials like:

- ***Jade:*** Known for soothing and calming properties.
- ***Rose Quartz:*** Popular for its cooling effect and connection to skincare.
- ***Obsidian:*** Best for relieving muscle tension.

Avoid: Cheap plastic tools or rough edges, as they could damage your skin. Invest in high-quality tools from reputable skincare brands.

Step 2: Prepare Your Skin

Preparing your skin correctly ensures smooth movement of the tool and prevents irritation. Follow these steps:

1. **Cleanse Your Face:** Wash your face with a gentle cleanser to remove dirt, oils, or makeup. Pat your skin dry with a clean towel.
2. **Apply Oil or Serum:** Use a generous layer of facial oil, serum, or cream to create a smooth glide. Choose oils based on your skin type:

- ***For Dry Skin:*** Opt for nourishing oils like argan or jojoba.
- ***For Sensitive Skin:*** Use calming blends like chamomile or aloe-infused oils.
- ***For Oily Skin:*** Lightweight oils such as grapeseed or squalane work best.

Make sure your skin feels slippery to avoid unnecessary friction or pulling.

Pro Tip: Warm the oil slightly by rubbing it between your palms before application to enhance relaxation.

Step 3: Begin Scraping with Proper Technique

Now that your tool is ready and the skin is prepped, it's time to start the Gua Sha ritual. Here's what to keep in mind:

Hold the Tool at the Correct Angle

The tool should be angled approximately 15 to 30 degrees against your skin while stroking. This prevents harsh gouging or scratching and ensures a smoother glide.

Apply Gentle but Firm Pressure

- Use light pressure for sensitive areas such as around the eyes.
- Apply slightly more firm strokes on the jawline and cheekbones.

General Rule: It should never hurt or cause pain. Consistency is key, not force.

Step-by-Step Instructions for Each Area

1. **Jawline and Chin**
   - Place the notched edge of your tool at the center of your chin, just above where your jaw meets.
   - Gently sweep outward toward your ear in slow, controlled movements.
   - Repeat 5-7 strokes on each side.

2. **Cheekbones**
   - Start at the side of your nose. Use the flat edge of the tool and glide upwards along your cheekbone, moving toward the temple.
   - Apply light pressure here to avoid pulling delicate skin.
   - Repeat 5-7 strokes on each cheek.

3. **Undereye Area**
   - With the flat, smooth edge, begin near the inner corner of your eye.
   - Gently move outward toward the temple using light pressure. Be extra delicate as this skin is thin.
   - Repeat 3-5 strokes on each side.

4. **Forehead**
   - Start at the center of your forehead, just above your brows.

- Glide the tool upward towards your hairline to lift the facial muscles.
- Gradually work outward toward your temples, following an upward motion.
- Repeat 5-7 strokes per section.

5. **Neck**
   - Starting at the base of your neck, use the long flat edge of the tool and glide upward toward your jawline.
   - Avoid scraping downwards as Gua Sha is believed to encourage upward lymphatic drainage.
   - Repeat 5-7 times on both sides.

Pro Tip: Always work in upward and outward motions. This not only helps with lymphatic drainage but also gives a natural lifting and sculpting effect.

Step 4: Final Touch - Cleaning and Cooling

Once your routine is complete:

1. Wash your face again gently with cold water to close the pores.
2. Wipe off any product residue and sterilize your Gua Sha tool with a gentle cleanser to maintain hygiene.

Optional Step: Place your Gua Sha tool in the fridge before use for an added cooling effect that helps with puffiness and redness.

Step 5: Moisturize and Relax

Seal the practice with a high-quality moisturizer or overnight mask. This locks in the benefits from the oils or serums used during the session.

Optional rituals to enhance the experience:

- Light a soothing candle or diffuse essential oils like lavender.
- Pair the session with a relaxing playlist or ambient music for a true self-care moment.

Pro Tip: If you're using Gua Sha at night, opt for richer moisturizers. For morning routines, pair it with a light, sun-protective skincare product.

Gua Sha offers a holistic approach to skincare that goes beyond external aesthetics. It relieves facial and muscular tension, promoting both physical beauty and inner calm. With consistency and the right techniques tailored to your needs, you'll uncover radiant and rejuvenated skin.

Creating a Gua Sha Routine

Starting a Gua Sha routine is simple, and it can easily become a relaxing part of your day. Here's how you can create a consistent practice that works for you:

1. **When to Do It**
   - *Morning Sessions:* Spend about 5–10 minutes to refresh your skin, reduce puffiness, and give your face a healthy glow.
   - *Evening Sessions:* Take 10–20 minutes to relax, ease muscle tension, and support your body's natural detox process before bed.
2. **How Often to Practice**
   - *For Skin Care and Glow:* 3–5 times a week is ideal to see improvements in tone and circulation.
   - *For Relaxation and Muscle Relief:* Use as needed when you feel tension—it could be daily or just a couple of times a week.
3. **Making It a Ritual**

Turn Gua Sha into "you time" by creating a calming environment. Here's how to make it extra special:

- *Music:* Play soft, soothing tunes to help you unwind.
- *Lighting:* Dim the lights or use candles for a cozy vibe.

- ***Aromatherapy:*** Try essential oils like lavender or eucalyptus to boost relaxation.

4. **Stick to a Routine**

    Choose a time that fits your schedule and make it a habit. You can do it while watching a show or as part of your skincare routine. With just a few minutes a day, you'll feel relaxed and refreshed.

By setting aside this time for self-care, Gua Sha can quickly become one of your favorite ways to relax and care for your body and mind.

DIY Gua Sha Recipes for Oils and Creams

Now that you know how to use a Gua Sha tool, let's take it a step further with some homemade recipes for oils and creams that can enhance your routine.

In this chapter, you'll find step-by-step recipes for soothing oils and creams designed for various skin types. Plus, we'll share practical tips on how to store and use your DIY creations safely, ensuring they remain fresh and effective.

Why Lubrication Matters for Gua Sha

Before we dive into the recipes, it's worth understanding why lubrication is so important for Gua Sha. Oils and creams help reduce friction, protecting your skin from irritation caused by the scraping motion of the tool. They also nourish the skin, deliver key nutrients, and boost the overall effectiveness of the practice by aiding in lymphatic drainage and circulation.

DIY Recipes for Gua Sha Oils

These basic oil recipes are infused with skin-loving ingredients and essential oils to create a silky base for your Gua Sha routine. Choose oils that suit your specific skin type for maximum results.

Anti-Inflammatory Calming Oil

Perfect for relieving redness and irritation, this blend offers anti-inflammatory properties and a soothing aroma. Ideal for sensitive skin or post-breakout care.

Ingredients:

- 2 tablespoons jojoba oil (a lightweight, non-comedogenic base oil)
- 3-5 drops lavender essential oil (anti-inflammatory and calming)
- 2 drops chamomile essential oil (soothes sensitive or red skin)
- Optional: 1 drop tea tree oil for mild antibacterial properties

Instructions:

1. Combine all the oils in a clean glass dropper bottle or jar.
2. Shake well to mix.
3. Apply 4-5 drops to your face or body before starting your Gua Sha session.

Hydrating Glow Oil (For Dry Skin)

This nourishing blend deeply hydrates and delivers a natural glow, perfect for dry or flaky skin.

Ingredients:

- 2 tablespoons sweet almond oil (rich in Vitamin E)
- 1 tablespoon argan oil (known for its intense hydration)
- 3 drops rose essential oil (hydrating and anti-aging)
- 2 drops frankincense essential oil (promotes cell turnover and skin healing)

Instructions:

1. Pour the carrier oils into a clean glass container.
2. Add the essential oils.
3. Mix thoroughly and store in a cool, dark place. Apply a small amount before your routine.

Balancing Facial Oil (For Oily or Acne-Prone Skin)

This lightweight formula nourishes without clogging pores, helping to balance sebum production and improve skin clarity.

Ingredients:

- 2 tablespoons grapeseed oil (light, fast-absorbing, and excellent for oily skin)
- 2 drops rosemary essential oil (reduces excess oil)
- 2 drops tea tree oil (antibacterial and clears blemishes)
- 2 drops geranium essential oil (balances skin's natural oil production)

Instructions:

1. Mix the grapeseed oil with the essential oils in a clean bottle.
2. Gently shake to combine.
3. Use sparingly—just a few drops are enough for your Gua Sha ritual.

Brightening Citrus Oil (For Dull or Uneven Skin Tone)

This refreshing blend energizes the skin while promoting a brighter, more even complexion. Grapefruit and orange essential oils are packed with antioxidants that help tackle dullness and reduce the appearance of dark spots.

Ingredients:

- 2 tablespoons jojoba oil (light and non-comedogenic, suitable for all skin types)
- 2 drops grapefruit essential oil (rich in vitamin C and brightens the skin)
- 2 drops sweet orange essential oil (uplifting scent and improves skin tone)
- 1 drop rosehip oil (targets hyperpigmentation and fine lines)

Instructions:

1. Pour jojoba and rosehip oils into a sterilized glass dropper bottle.
2. Add the essential oils into the mix.
3. Give the bottle a gentle shake to combine all ingredients.
4. Apply 4-5 drops to your face and neck before starting your Gua Sha routine, avoiding sun exposure immediately after due to citrus oil sensitivity.

Soothing Recovery Oil (For Irritated or Post-Sunburn Skin)

Designed for skin that needs extra care and healing, this blend reduces irritation and promotes repair with calming essential oils. It's perfect for sunburns, windburn, or post-inflammatory redness.

Ingredients:

- 2 tablespoons aloe vera gel (hydrating and soothing base)
- 1 tablespoon calendula oil (known for its healing properties)
- 3 drops chamomile essential oil (anti-inflammatory and calming)
- 2 drops lavender essential oil (reduces redness and irritation)
- 1 drop peppermint essential oil (adds a cooling sensation)

Instructions:

1. Combine aloe vera gel and calendula oil in a small mixing bowl.
2. Add the essential oils and stir until well blended.
3. Transfer the mix to a pump bottle or jar for easy application.
4. Apply a light layer to clean skin before your Gua Sha massage.

With these DIY Gua Sha oil recipes, you can tailor your skincare routine to your specific needs, whether it's hydration, calming, or brightening. Simple to make and packed with nourishing ingredients, these blends enhance your Gua Sha practice for healthier, glowing skin.

DIY Recipes for Gua Sha Creams

When oils feel too heavy or you prefer a silky finish, creams tailored to your skin type offer a great alternative.

Gentle Chamomile Cream (For Sensitive or Red-Prone Skin)

This handcrafted cream repairs your skin barrier while offering a smooth glide for facial Gua Sha.

Ingredients:

- 2 tablespoons shea butter (hydrates and soothes inflammation)
- 1 tablespoon aloe vera gel (calms redness and irritation)
- 3 drops chamomile essential oil
- 3 drops calendula oil (healing and soothing for sensitive skin)

Instructions:

1. Melt shea butter gently in a double boiler.
2. Stir in aloe vera gel and mix thoroughly.
3. Add essential oils, stir, and transfer to a small jar.
4. Allow the cream to cool and solidify before use.

Anti-Aging Rosehip Cream (For Mature Skin)

Rosehip oil rejuvenates skin while this luxurious cream deeply moisturizes.

Ingredients:

- 2 tablespoons cocoa butter (rich in antioxidants)
- 1 tablespoon rosehip oil (reduces fine lines)
- 3 drops frankincense essential oil
- 2 drops ylang-ylang essential oil (promotes skin elasticity)

Instructions:

1. Melt cocoa butter in a double boiler.
2. Add rosehip oil and essential oils.
3. Transfer to a jar and stir occasionally as it sets to maintain a creamy texture.
4. Store in a cool, dry place and use as needed.

Lightweight Green Tea Gel (For Oily or Acne-Prone Skin)

This refreshing gel provides a cooling, matte finish, perfect for skin that needs hydration without heaviness.

Ingredients:

- 2 tablespoons aloe vera gel (hydrating and calming)
- 1 teaspoon green tea extract (antioxidant-rich and purifying)
- 2 drops tea tree oil
- 2 drops peppermint essential oil (cools and refreshes skin)

Instructions:

1. Combine all ingredients in a small dish.
2. Mix until smooth and store in an airtight container.
3. Apply a thin layer before your Gua Sha session.

Brightening Vitamin C Cream (For Dull or Uneven Skin Tone)

This lightweight cream combines ingredients known for their brightening properties, leaving the skin refreshed and glowing. Perfect for tackling dullness and uneven skin tones.

Ingredients:

- 2 tablespoons shea butter (nourishes and repairs skin)
- 1 teaspoon vitamin C powder (brightens and evens out skin tone)
- 1 tablespoon rose water (hydrates and soothes)
- 3 drops orange essential oil (antioxidant-rich and uplifting)

Instructions:

1. Melt the shea butter in a double boiler over low heat until smooth.
2. Remove from heat and mix in the rose water slowly, stirring constantly to ensure emulsification.
3. Add the vitamin C powder and stir until fully dissolved.
4. Blend in the orange essential oil.
5. Pour the cream into a small clean jar and allow it to cool and set.
6. Apply a thin layer before a Gua Sha session to brighten and hydrate.

Deep Hydration Avocado Cream (For Extremely Dry or Flaky Skin)

This ultra-rich cream is designed to deeply moisturize and repair the driest of skin types. Avocado oil and natural butters ensure long-lasting hydration.

Ingredients:

- 2 tablespoons mango butter (ultra-hydrating and reparative)
- 1 tablespoon avocado oil (rich in vitamins A, D, and E)
- 1 teaspoon glycerin (locks in moisture)
- 2 drops lavender essential oil (calms and soothes dryness)

Instructions:

1. Gently melt the mango butter in a double boiler until it becomes liquid.
2. Slowly stir in the avocado oil and glycerin, ensuring all ingredients are well combined.
3. Add the lavender essential oil and mix thoroughly.
4. Transfer to a sterilized jar and allow it to cool at room temperature.
5. Use a small amount to prep extremely dry areas before your Gua Sha routine.

These DIY Gua Sha creams and gels are simple to make and tailored to suit your skin's unique needs. Whether you're looking for hydration, brightness, or a lightweight finish, these recipes offer natural, effective solutions for your skincare routine.

Tips for Storing and Using DIY Products

Homemade oils and creams can offer a luxurious experience, but proper storage and care are crucial to maintain their quality and safety.

- *Use Clean Containers:* Ensure all jars and bottles are sterilized before storing your creations. This prevents contamination and extends shelf life.
- *Store in a Cool, Dark Place:* Heat and sunlight can degrade essential oils and carrier oils. Keep your products in a bathroom cabinet or cosmetic fridge.
- *Label and Date Your Products:* Homemade products don't always have preservatives, so use them within 30-60 days. Adding a label with the creation date ensures you keep track.
- *Patch Test First:* Before applying a new oil or cream, test a small amount on a patch of skin (e.g., behind your ear) to check for any allergic reactions.
- *Avoid Water Contact:* Keep your fingers dry when scooping creams to prevent growth of bacteria or mold.

No single recipe fits everyone. Experiment with these blends to find the one that best suits your personal skin type and goals. The beauty of DIY is that you can tweak recipes as you go—adding ingredients that work wonders for your skin or adjusting essential oil concentrations based on your preferences.

By incorporating these lubricants into your Gua Sha routine, not only will your tools glide effortlessly, but your skin will also soak up the nourishing benefits, leaving you relaxed, rejuvenated, and radiant.

Gua Sha and Graston Technique

You could be familiar with Gua Sha and the Graston Technique, but you could be curious about how the two approaches are comparable to one another. The Graston Technique and the Gua Sha method are both types of treatment that include the use of instruments to massage the patient's skin.

The practice of Gua Sha, which is a kind of traditional Chinese medicine, consists of massaging the skin with a blunt instrument. Scrape or rub is what the Chinese character Gua implies, whereas Sha refers to sand or rigidity. Gua Sha is performed to release any congestion or stagnation that may be present beneath the skin. This may aid in the reduction of pain, enhance circulation, and reduce inflammation.

Instrument-assisted soft tissue mobilization is the basis of the Graston Technique, which is a type of treatment (IASTM). IASTM is a form of therapy that involves massaging the patient's skin with specialized devices. Scar tissue and adhesions under the skin can be broken up with the assistance of the devices. This may assist in the treatment of pain, the improvement of range of motion, and the reduction of inflammation.

Some parallels can be drawn between the Graston Technique and the Gua Sha technique. In each of these treatments, instruments are used to massage the patient's skin. Both of these treatments can help relieve pain, as well as enhance circulation and bring down inflammatory levels.

Gua Sha and the Graston Technique have key differences despite their similarities. Gua Sha, rooted in traditional Chinese medicine, has been used for centuries as a healing method. The Graston Technique, developed in the 1990s, is a modern approach. Gua Sha is performed by practitioners trained in Chinese medicine, while the Graston Technique can be done by any healthcare professional trained in Instrument-Assisted Soft Tissue Mobilization (IASTM).

Conclusion

Thank you for joining us on this in-depth exploration of Gua Sha! By now, you've gained a comprehensive understanding of this ancient Chinese practice—its rich history, practical tools, techniques, and the incredible benefits it can offer your overall wellness and beauty routine.

Gua Sha is not just any practice; it's a testament to the wisdom of Traditional Chinese Medicine. This holistic approach aligns beauty, health, and energy into one seamless ritual that you can easily incorporate into your life. Whether you're seeking relief from muscle tension, brighter skin, or a moment of peace from your busy day, Gua Sha has something for everyone. It works with your body, not against it, gently encouraging self-healing and balance.

The beauty of Gua Sha lies in its simplicity. You don't need a spa appointment or expensive products to enjoy its effects. With the right tool and a few minutes, you can create a soothing, self-care ritual right at home. From improving lymphatic drainage for puffiness to rejuvenating skin tone or relieving deep-seated tension in your back, Gua Sha offers profound benefits for both body and mind.

But remember, the secret to maximizing the benefits of Gua Sha is consistency and proper technique. Like any self-care practice, your results will improve over time as you become more familiar with the tools and movements. Be patient with yourself, and allow the practice to become a comforting ritual in your routine. Even devoting just 10 minutes a few times a week can make a difference. Over time, you'll not only see improvements in your skin and physical well-being but may also notice a calmer, more centered state of mind.

Equally important as consistency is safety. Always listen to your body—use the right amount of pressure, avoid sensitive or injured areas, and ensure your tools are clean and high-quality. If you're new to Gua Sha or have any health concerns, consulting with a healthcare professional or trained practitioner is a key step to ensuring a safe and effective experience.

The magic of Gua Sha comes not just from its physical benefits but also from the intention you bring to it. Think of each stroke as a way to care for yourself fully—nurturing your skin, boosting your energy, and grounding your emotions. By treating Gua Sha as more than just a routine but a mindful act of self-love, you invite balance and harmony into your life.

Now, it's your turn to take this knowledge and apply it. Begin your Gua Sha practice, experiment with oils and tools, and explore what this time-honored method can do for you. Whether it becomes a morning glow booster or an evening relaxation ritual, Gua Sha is a gentle reminder to slow down and reconnect with your well-being.

Here's to your next step toward wellness, beauty, and balance—one stroke at a time. You're not just following an ancient tradition; you're cultivating your path to self-care in a world that often asks for more than we can give. Thank you for completing this guide, and may your Gua Sha practice bring lightness, transformation, and peace to your days.

FAQ

Can you tell me about gua sha?

A method of traditional Chinese medicine known as gua sha includes using a smooth, blunt object to scrape the surface of the skin in a circular motion. It is believed that the technique will increase circulation by breaking up stagnation in the body, which will then facilitate healing. Gua sha is usually employed as a treatment for aches, inflammation, and even the common cold.

What is the procedure for gua sha?

The jade stone or ceramic spoon that is often used in gua sha therapy is an example of a tool that is both smooth and blunt. After applying oil to the patient's skin to lubricate it, the practitioner will scrape a tool across the patient's skin in a manner that is both hard and gentle. The scraping shouldn't be uncomfortable, although it's possible that some bruising will take place.

Can you tell me about the advantages of using gua sha?

It is believed that gua sha may enhance circulation, boost healing, and significantly cut down on pain and inflammation. Additionally, it is believed that gua sha can strengthen the immune system and assist in the treatment of illnesses like the common cold and influenza.

Does gua sha have any potential negative effects?

After receiving a gua sha treatment, you can have some bruising, but this is usually just brief and will go away in a few days at the most. It is essential to refrain from rubbing the skin too roughly since this might result in an injury if not avoided. Gua sha is not dangerous for the vast majority of individuals when it is done properly.

How frequently should I have gua sha treatments?

The frequency of gua sha treatments will change from person to person according to what that person requires. Some people may benefit from having treatments performed once a week, while others would simply require treatments on an as-needed basis. When determining the frequency with which gua sha should be administered, it is critical to seek the advice of an experienced practitioner.

How long does a treatment with gua sha typically last?

The duration of a gua sha treatment typically ranges from ten to fifteen minutes; however, the amount of time may change based on the requirements of the individual.

Is gua sha a useful method for treating the face?

It is believed that regular use of gua sha can assist to enhance complexion as well as lessen the appearance of wrinkles on the face. In addition to this, it is stated that gua sha can assist alleviate tension headaches as well as neck discomfort.

Who shouldn't have gua sha treatment?

Because of their medical problems or other circumstances, certain people should not have the gua sha treatment. These individuals include those who are pregnant, those who are taking medications that thin the blood, as well as those who have open wounds or illnesses.

References and Helpful Links

Life, S. (2020, August 25). Gua Sha 101 : All about how to use the Gua Sha tool. Sublime Life. https://sublimelife.in/blogs/sublime-stories/gua-sha-101-everything-you-need-to-know-about-how-to-use-a-gua-sha

Ewe, K., & Ewe, K. (2024, August 9). Does Gua Sha work? What two weeks of trying the beauty trend did to my face. VICE. https://www.vice.com/en/article/g5ggv7/gua-sha-benefits-beauty-skincare-trend

Wang, S. (2021, June 26). Gua sha Step-by-Step Tutorial. La Coéss. https://www.lacoess.com/blogs/news/gua-sha-step-by-step-tutorial

Quinn, D. (2021, January 22). How to use Gua sha for tension, puffiness, and lymphatic drainage. Healthline. https://www.healthline.com/health/beauty-skin-care/how-to-use-gua-sha

Imelda, J. D. (n.d.). Got a cold? In coin rubbing Indonesians trust. The Conversation. http://theconversation.com/got-a-cold-in-coin-rubbing-indonesians-trust-79270

Baruah, N. (2024, March 18). Is Gua Sha the newest beauty self-care tool? We think so! Lifestyle Asia India. https://www.lifestyleasia.com/ind/beauty-grooming/skincare/is-gua-sha-the-newest-beauty-self-care-tool-we-think-so/

The art of Gua Sha, or scraping therapy. (2019, December 2). Lifemark. https://www.lifemark.ca/blog-post/art-gua-sha-or-scraping-therapy

Noble, B. &. (n.d.). GUA SHA: AN ANCIENT THERAPY FOR CONTEMPORARY ILLNESSES: An Ancient Therapy for Contemporary Illnesses|Hardcover. Barnes & Noble. https://www.barnesandnoble.com/w/gua-sha-kai-wen-tang/1133363529

Understanding the role of the kidney. (n.d.). https://www.euyansang.com/en_US/tcm%3A-understanding-the-role-of-the-kidney/eystcmorgans2.html

Nashville Hip Institute at TOA, Preservation, Reconstruction & Sports Medicine. (2021, October 19). IASTM. Nashville Hip Institute at TOA | Thomas Byrd MD. https://nashvillehip.org/iastm/

Why gua sha is good for you. (2021, June 14). Cleveland Clinic Health Essentials. https://health.clevelandclinic.org/why-gua-sha-might-be-good-for-you/.

www.ingramcontent.com/pod-product-compliance
Lightning Source LLC
LaVergne TN
LVHW012030060526
838201LV00061B/4534